Praise for Learning to Walk in the Dark

"Every now and then, a book stops you in your tracks, and *Learning to Walk in the Dark* by Viv Grant is one such book—a work of pure joy and wisdom. Drawing from her battle with cancer, Viv shares how, during her season of darkness, she turned to painting as her light and overcame adversity with courage and grace.

This is a book the world has been waiting for—transformative, hopeful, and deeply moving. I'm truly grateful for this gift and am sure you'll enjoy the pilgrimage too.

Dr Anita Devi

"My heart aches at the exquisite tenderness and wisdom suffused throughout *Learning to Walk in the Dark*. Viv Grant has not only traversed her inner landscape with courage, compassion and commitment, she has translated each chapter of her journey in such a way, that the reader is resourced to explore their darkest depths with strength, reassurance and gentle curiosity.

Whether you have just received a frightening diagnosis, have been struggling with a chronic condition, physical or mental; or whether you are simply exhausted by the egoic noise invading your life, *Walking in the Dark* will inspire you to bravely embark inward.

With moving, earthy paintings to call you home to your own soul and alchemical reflections to guide your path, this book will support your journey of deep connection to your inner world, enabling you to live more authentically in the outer world.

Viv's warm glow of compassionate guidance will help you voyage through your own darkness into a new dawn. A dynamic creative journal for anyone willing to respond to the calling of Stillness."

Kathryn Lovewell, Author, Self-Compassion Teacher.

In this beautiful book, Viv takes her reader on a journey through life's downs and ups. She shows vulnerability, courage, and strength in describing her journey onto resolution and wellness, following diagnosis of serious illness. It is a unique fusion of inspirational quotes, advice from ancient and modern times bound up with gorgeous thought-provoking original art.

In this powerful book, Viv imparts her wisdom and knowledge of leadership, whilst sharing the insights and different perspectives her cancer diagnosis gave her. It is clear that sometimes life and fate make choices for you, and you have no choice but to go along on the journey. This book will be a companion to you for the times in your life where you need to stop and rest or to reset. It will help you to realise that sometimes there is an alternative path which needs to be travelled.

Dr Susan Davis, Associate Professor, Cardiff Metropolitan University.

'For anyone who has felt isolated by the weight of leadership challenges, the masterful Viv Grant has provided us all with an empathetic, empowering journey toward self-discovery.
Viv eloquently reminds us that true leadership often begins in vulnerability, and by accepting the dark, we allow new light and strength to emerge.
A must-read for leaders seeking a profound, authentic path to personal and professional renewal.'

Lucy Coy, Co-Founder Headteacher Chat

Learning to walk in the dark is both deeply moving and uplifting and it is also so good for your soul.

I immediately felt that I was on a journey with Viv as she talked us through her cancer diagnosis and how she came to terms with what lay ahead. The ability to be vulnerable whilst also being hopeful is such a wonderful skill as it invites the reader to also dig deep and reflect on areas of their lives that may have been challenging.

What I particularly liked about this book is how Viv has used art as a powerful expression of emotions which really bring each section to life. It reminded me that we should never underestimate the power of words coupled with art.

Before the book concludes, *Homecoming* offers brightness and hope and an opportunity to reflect on how much your soul will have been nourished.

Learning to walk in the dark is more than a book and more than a journal, it is a combination of powerful words and artwork that make this a truly special read.

Evelyn Forde MBE

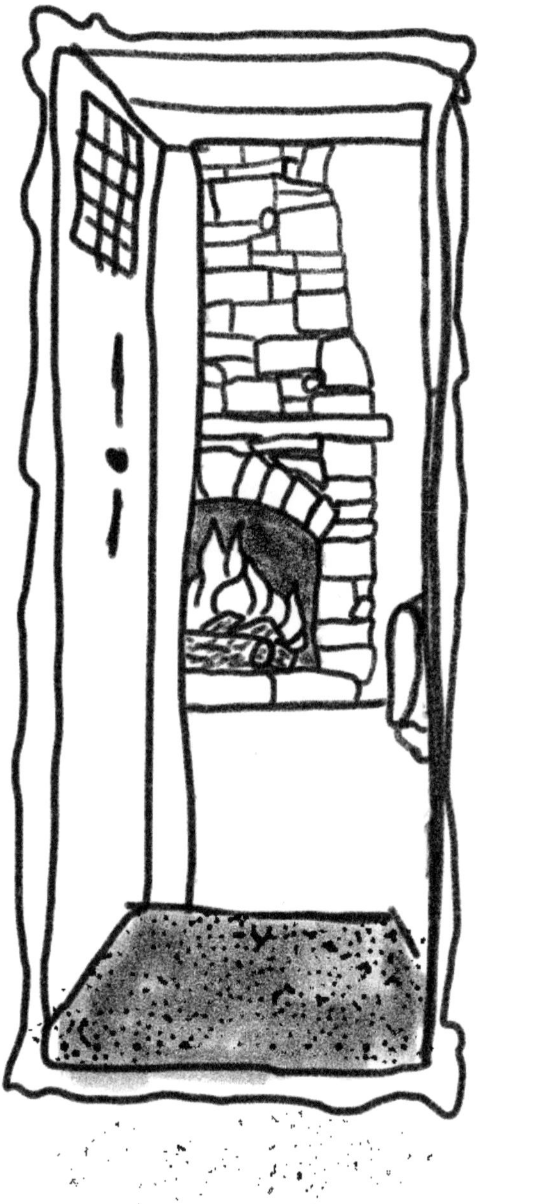

The Guest House

"This being human is a guest house.
Every morning a new arrival.
A joy, a depression, a meanness,
some momentary awareness comes
as an unexpected visitor.
Welcome and entertain them all!
Even if they're a crowd of sorrows,
who violently sweep your house
empty of its furniture,
still, treat each guest honorably.
They may be clearing you out
for some new delight.
The dark thought, the shame, the malice,
meet them at the door laughing,
and invite them in.
Be grateful for whoever comes,
because each has been sent
as a guide from beyond."

Jalaluddin Rumi

Learning to Walk in the Dark

This edition first published 2025

ISBN: 978-1-0369-0786-0

A CIP catalogue record for this book is available from the British Library.

Integrity Coaching Ltd
Unit D228, Parkhall Business Centre
62 Tritton Road
London SE21 8DE
United Kingdom
Website: www.integritycoaching.co.uk

Publishing Location:
Published in the United Kingdom by **Integrity Coaching Ltd**

Cover design, Viv Grant & Izzy Spitz
Original Artwork, Viv Grant
Pen and Ink illustrations, Izzy Spitz

Printed and bound in the United Kingdom

First edition: January 2025

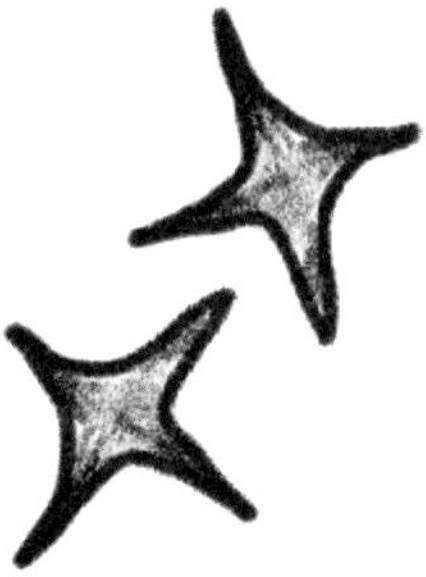

For Lauren and Eisha, two of the brightest stars,

and fellow night guides,

Tris, Isaac and Curtis-Ray

CONTENTS

PART 1: The Descent

PART 2: The Darkness

PART 3: The New Dawn

HOMECOMING

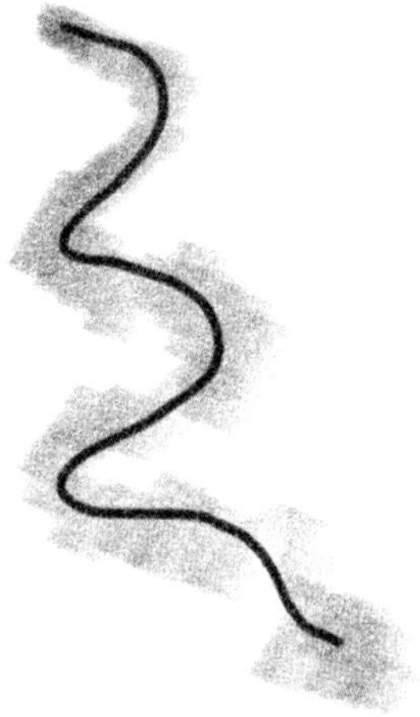

INTRODUCTION

Answering the Call to Growth

As human beings, there will inevitably be moments along life's way when the light seems to dim, and we find ourselves adrift, unsure of our direction. These are the times when we stumble, wander and feel lost. When we are beckoned to traverse unexpected paths and darkness becomes our companion and guide.

While daunting, these journeys can often serve as invitations to embark on a profound voyage of self-discovery, what Jung termed the individuation process. Regrettably, many fail to recognise this call, unaware of the psychological, emotional, and spiritual metamorphosis awaiting us as we age. Consequently, we stumble in our quest for solid ground, grasping futilely at external anchors instead of seeking solace and answers from within.

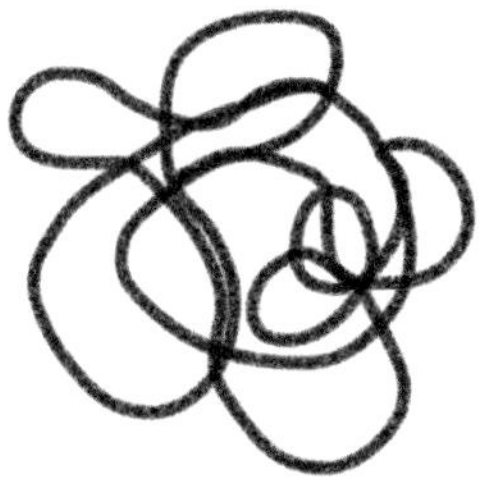

Navigating the Darkness

The ancients suggest that in these moments of darkness, if we remain still and patient, we may discover that we are not truly lost but rather undergoing a type of soul initiation. It's as if our very essence is seeking a new path forward. Though it may not feel like it at first, these dark times often herald the emergence of something positive and transformative into the light of our consciousness. As we journey through the darkest of nights, confronting our pain, worries, and fears head-on, we begin to discern glimpses of our true selves and the unique purpose of our lives.

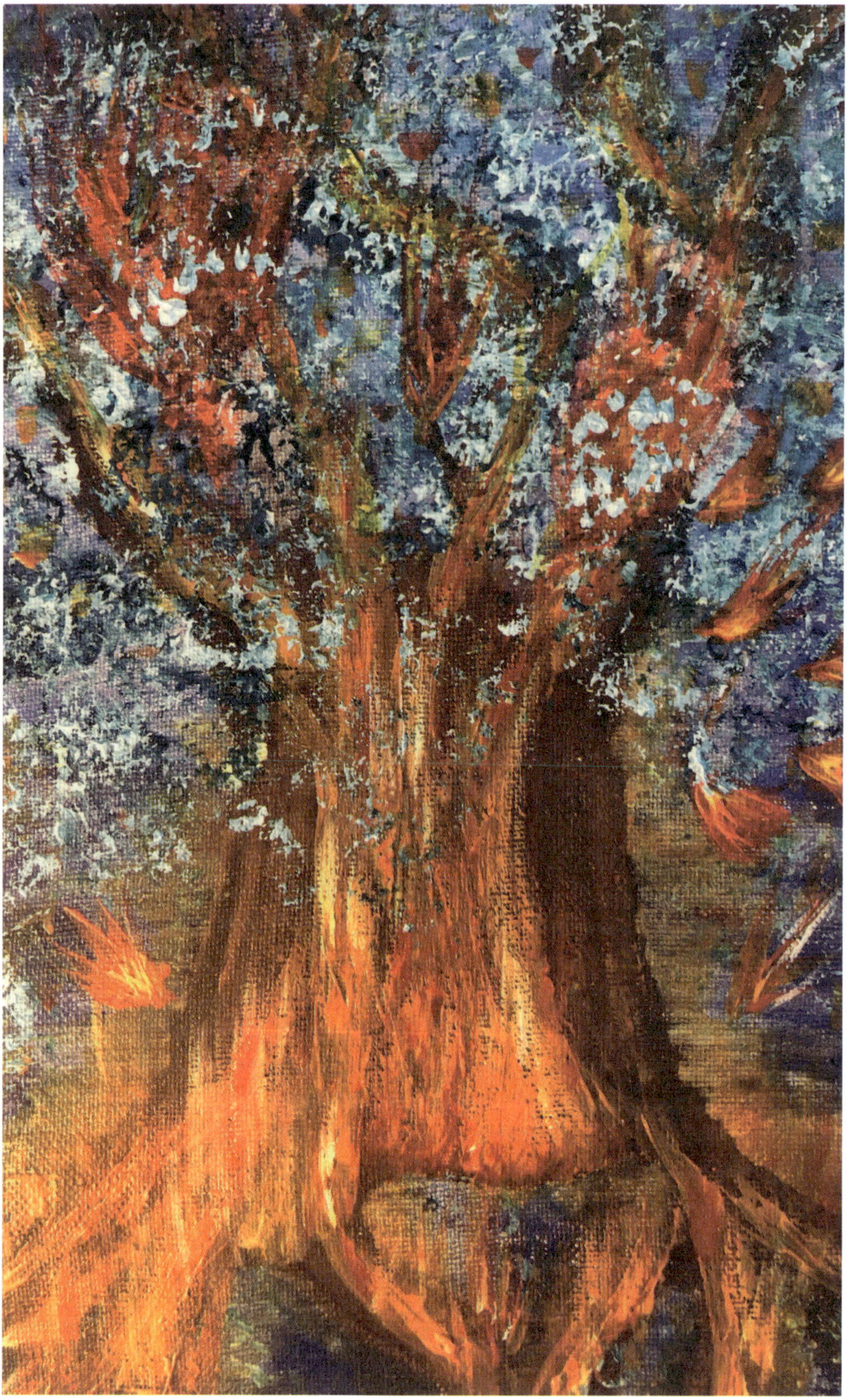

"Just as after a devastating forest fire, the seeds of a new forest wait in the soil, it helps us to remember the archetype of destruction/creation: new life arrives only after the end of the old way and grief is a necessary part of any deep transformation."

Bill Plotkin
(Wildnerness Guide and Eco-Depth Psychologist)

Finding New Ways to Walk in the Dark

Countless volumes have been penned on the transformative potential of the soul's journey when we experience significant life challenges. Yet, in my experience, when we travel through the darkest of nights, we have scant energy to sift through thousands of words in search of solace and understanding.

Intellectualism, processing, and rationalisation, while valuable in their own right, often fall short in the shadowy realms of the soul. As Thomas Moore, author of "Dark Nights of the Soul," aptly puts it, they are but "daytime biases." What we truly need are our nocturnal senses, those innate capacities to navigate the darkened corridors of our inner world. Unfortunately, many of us find these faculties underdeveloped due to our collective aversion to solitude, the ability to be at ease in our own company and when necessary, to use the time to abide with the darkness, be still and sit in both silence and reverence with our fears and vulnerabilities.

Hence, this book adopts a different approach.

It is not an academic treatise on the journey of the soul. It is not concerned with right or wrong or presenting arguments for and against. It is only concerned with helping you to identify what feels true and right for you.

Consider it more of a reflective journal, a companion for the journey you are on. It beckons you to "Learn to Walk in the Dark" by employing imagery and enquiry as primary tools for reflection. It invites you to imagine, look with new eyes, adopt a beginner's mind and reflect from the depths of your own being.

Discovering Beauty in the Darkness

It has been my own experience (and perhaps you have found the same, too) that navigating the darkness is a multifaceted journey, one that can paradoxically be both complex and surprisingly simple, beautiful and serene if we allow it to be.

However, embracing the darkness can be challenging. Forgotten are the sacred memories of our time cocooned within our mothers' wombs, where darkness nurtured us. From a young age, we're taught to fear the dark. How many of us only felt safe enough to sleep with the light on, believing in our innocence that the light warded off the monsters that lurked in our dreams or under our beds? For how many of us did these monsters (real or imagined) stay with us well into adulthood? For how many of us has it taken a strange and unexpected turn of events for us to have the courage to finally face the dark and learn not to be afraid but instead to discover that an invitation awaits.

An invitation to accept the wonders and secrets that it holds. It's almost as though we need to be reminded that darkness, just as Mother Nature demonstrates, can be a harbinger of new life and a season of rest and renewal. If only we could allow ourselves to be still long enough and let nature/life take its course.

Letting Go of the Familiar

Yet amidst the cacophony of daily life, our fears, worries and self-doubt can obscure the sacred nature of any night journey we might find ourselves on. We can so easily miss the signs, fail to notice the glimmers of light in the darkness, and cling to what feels safe and familiar, unaware that these old habits only serve to keep us stuck. To truly navigate the darkness, we must release these familiar moorings and embrace new ways of being.

Embracing Uncertainty

It was my own journey with cancer that taught me at a much deeper level how to walk in the dark, how to sit with uncertainty and allow a more profound wisdom to emerge. As a seasoned coach, I have often journeyed alongside others going through their own 'dark night of the soul'. Having been through a fair few dark nights of my own, I felt that I had the capacity, empathy and wherewithal to help my clients find the proverbial light at the end of the tunnel. However, with my cancer diagnosis, there was a fundamental shift in my comprehension of the process of individuation. I was taken to depths within my own being that I had never encountered before and truth be known, the experience rocked me to my core.

However, as the shadows began to recede and I found myself more at home in the dark, I began to understand more fully the words of Quaker author and social activist Parker J Palmer. Words that had initially been gifted to me as a beautiful wall hanging by a dear colleague in the aftermath of Covid and the murder of George Floyd. When I'd found myself facing some very painful emotions and experienced an internal devastation of sorts.

Palmer says;

“By choosing integrity, I
become more whole,
But wholeness does not mean
perfection.
It means becoming more real
by acknowledging
the whole of who I am.
It means embracing
brokenness as an integral
part of life.
Knowing this gives me hope
that human wholeness
Mine, yours, ours – need not
be a utopian dream
If we can use devastation as a
seedbed for new life.”

These words spoke volumes to me then. Following my cancer diagnosis, their meaning and significance for my life became even more pronounced.

A Great Complexity of Emotion

When I received my diagnosis, I felt like I was living someone else's life, half-expecting a call to tell me they'd confused my patient records.

However, as one doctor's appointment led to another, followed by referrals and visits to the Royal Marsden (the leading cancer hospital in London), the reality set in. No mistake had been made; it was indeed me, Viv Grant, who had Uterine Serous Carcinoma (A rare cancer, predominate in women of colour), and it was I who needed a hysterectomy and possibly additional treatment to prevent a recurrence.

The late Irish Poet and Philosopher John O'Donohue said that when we stand at a threshold, "A great complexity of emotion comes alive." This was indeed true for me. I experienced sadness, confusion, fear, and a whole range of other emotions in between.

As I gradually came to terms with the truth of my situation, I knew that the question I needed to grapple with upon encountering this unexpected threshold was not just "What do I need to do?" Yes, research and seeking information about my specific cancer were necessary. Still, an equally, if not more crucial, question emerged – a question I've often posed to clients facing crises: "Who do I need to be?"

Finding an Answer

Once again, the writings of John O'Donohue helped me find an answer to this question. In his Blessing "For a Friend, on the Arrival of Illness", he writes.

> "May you find
> in yourself
> A courageous
> hospitality
> Towards what
> is difficult,
> Painful and
> unknown."

"How do I summon a courageous hospitality towards a cancer diagnosis? How do I extend a courageous hospitality to a body now marked by major surgery? How do I offer such hospitality to the wounds, hurts, and confusion that envelop me on almost every level?" For a while, these questions circled around in my head. My instinctive response was to rely on my intellect to accumulate knowledge about my diagnosis and take action. However, something on the fringes of my awareness whispered, "Viv, thinking, reading, and researching alone won't carry you through this."

I now recognise that whisper, that gentle nudge at the edge of my consciousness, as the voice of my soul. It wasn't until I quieted the voice of my ego – the fear, the worries, the "what ifs" – that I formed a deeper connection with myself and found answers through silence and a huge amount of self-compassion. I needed to let go, if only momentarily, of my role as Viv Grant, Director of Integrity Coaching. I needed to cry, or rather, to sob! I needed to withdraw from the world. I needed to embrace the winter of my life and explore the elemental nature of my being. I needed to embrace vulnerability and confront the darkness and its accompanying shadows.

Finding Light in the Dark

In the darkness, I found solace in painting. A true gift of my own dark night of the soul. Painting was not something that I had ever done before. Not even as a hobby or an interest when I was at school. I could admire art and the work of others, but not for one moment had I ever considered myself an 'artist'. Yet, it was when I was most fearful and found no comfort from the protestations of my ego, through the sheer exhaustion of trying to keep my worry at bay, that I was forced to be still. To fall into the deep, luminous space of my inner being and listen to the soft whispers from within. Each of us possesses our own unique soul language, which becomes especially important during times of struggle and challenge. It is this sacred language that we must learn to understand and appreciate if we are to navigate the dark with grace and resilience.

My paintings appeared to depict my inner world, what was occurring deep within me as my rational mind stepped down from its usual position of dominance and allowed my soul, my deep inner intuition, to take centre stage.

Most of my paintings were of trees, roots buried deep within the earth. I felt they were symbolic of the deep alchemical work that happens hidden out of sight in winter. A time when the cold and often bleak and barren landscape can lead us to believe that everything has died. The trees look forlorn, no longer resplendent in the colours of the preceding seasons. But if you look closely, as I learned during this time, the trees are, in fact, alive with the promise of spring. Even in the midst of winter, buds are already beginning to appear!

So, my paintings became expressions of hope, reminders to trust in the wisdom of my soul and the perennial lessons that nature's rhythms and cycles provide us. It was clear: I was not to be afraid of the dark.

The dark is where growth happens, where new perspectives can

be found. The dark is where nature nurtures the tentative beginnings of new life.

Nature knows best, and my soul did, too.

Had I not taken such a steadfast inward glance, I very much doubt whether I would have found the treasure hidden deep within some of my darkest moments and indeed, this book might not even exist!

Katherine May, the author of the Sunday Times Bestseller "Wintering," says of this alchemical season, "Wintering brings about some of the most profound and insightful moments of our human experience." With each passing day, I am beginning to understand more and more exactly what she means.

This is your journey, too!

It was only after some time had passed and I looked back at the canvasses that I had painted during my recovery that I realised that they depicted the archetypal journey of the soul—a journey that we all must undertake and repeat with varying degrees of intensity at different stages in our lives. It is a journey marked by upheaval, by the disruption of the familiar and the emergence of something new. We must learn to traverse this liminal space, embracing the unknown and eventually emerging transformed. Rarely is the transformation swift. It is a process that requires us to develop a profound relationship with our own vulnerability and a new sense of self as we emerge from the darkness into the light.

Unfortunately, our society often fails to recognise the profound nature of the soul's journey, leading many to numb themselves to the inevitable pain of life. We fail to realise that this pain is a summons—a call to become more fully ourselves and to discover how we might better serve the greater good.

“Knowing how to be solitary is central to the art of living”

bell hooks
(Author, theorist, educator and social critic)

How To Get The Most Out Of This Book

If you find yourself holding this book, it may be because you are undergoing your own dark night of the soul and seeking a non-traditional path forward. One that doesn't seek to bypass the inevitable pain but instead invites you to find a way to sit with discomfort and embrace all it has to teach you.

This book is designed to assist you on your journey. Divided into three sections that capture three specific stages of the Soul's Journey—The Descent, The Darkness, and The New Dawn—it offers a series of paintings that emerged during my own recovery from cancer surgery. I hope that these paintings will serve as a mirror, reflecting the stages of transformation and offering inspiration for your own journey.

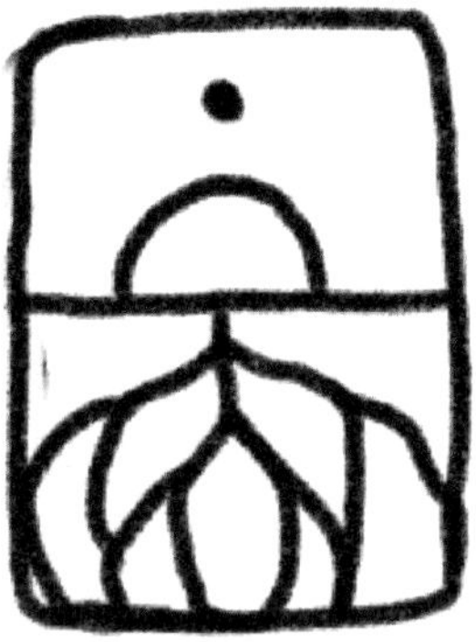

Reflection and Integration

At the end of each section, you'll find a specific invitation:

- At **the descent**, you are invited to **create a safe space**.
-During **the darkness**, you are invited to **welcome the night.**
-At the arrival of **the new dawn**, you are invited to **step outside.**

Each invitation has been designed to help you engage with questions about five core qualities: Curiosity, Commitment, Courage, Compassion, and Connection. These ways for engaging with life became intimate travel companions for me during this particular dark night. I consider these to be the five Cs of inner leadership, a capacity we all require when navigating life's shadowlands.

The 5 C's: An Overview

1. Curiosity: The capacity to engage with questions that cause you to look beyond the surface of your life

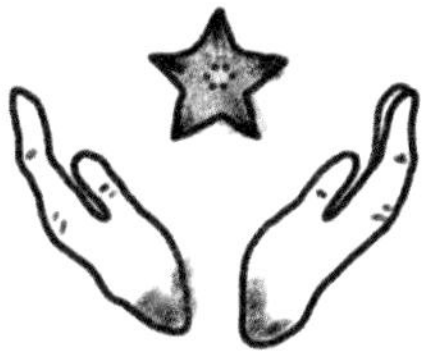

2. Commitment: The capacity to commit to 'The road less travelled' and develop new norms and ways of being that serve the greater whole and move beyond competition and individualism

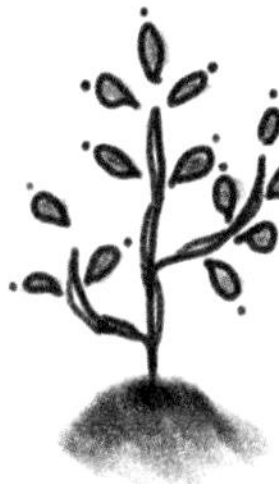

3. Courage: The capacity to embrace vulnerability and personal and cultural shadows to develop psychological maturity and wisdom that underpin good leadership (personally and professionally)

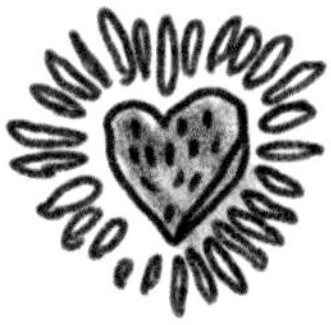

4. Compassion: The capacity to treat oneself with understanding and self-compassion as old habits are let loose and replaced by new generative ones.

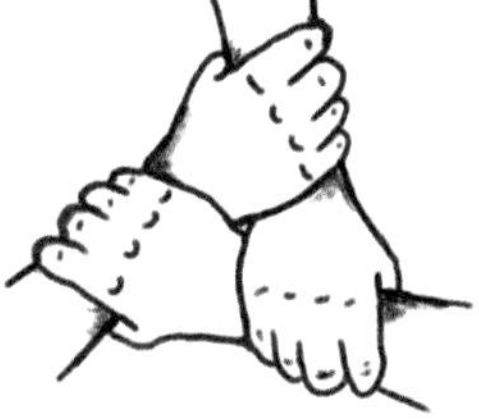

5. Connection: The capacity to build deeper relationships with self, others and the planet

Through my journey, I realised that these qualities will ask you different questions at each stage of your journey. They will challenge you to delve deeper into your own soul's quest and to integrate your experiences into your life.

An On-Going Conversation

When you arrive at the relevant sections in this book, I encourage you to devote quality time to reflecting on your responses to the questions and prompts. Resist the urge to answer them all at once. Learning to walk in the dark is not a process that can be rushed. It needs time—time to allow for the maturation of new sensibilities that will inevitably arise within you as you learn to navigate your new internal landscape. Rushing will only circumvent the process and you may never fully discover the treasure that is yours to be found as you learn to make sense of your own night passage.

Seek to be in a constant yet gentle conversation with the questions and you will find a rich dialogue emerging to help you navigate the way ahead. As you do, you'll also discover the light that shines within you—the light that will guide you, as you too, learn to walk in the dark.

Winter

will take you

by surprise.

The Descent

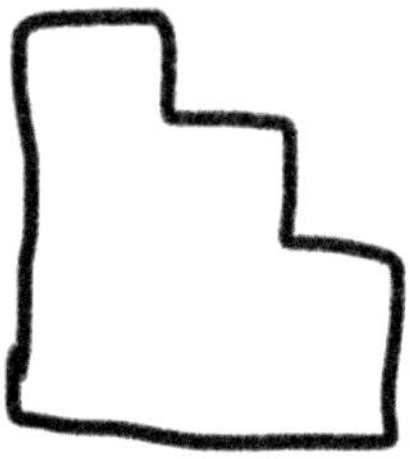

Winter will take you by surprise.
And the darkness, too
A descent to depths unknown
In silence, you stand alone
The night claims you as its own

The Darkness

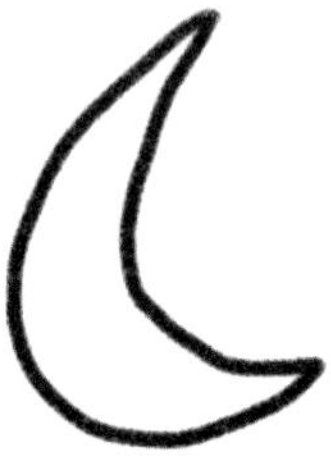

A slow revealing of the sacred nature of your descent
An inner purging of all that once felt so real
Love opens the doorway to your heart
Revealing buried treasure deep within
Spring hints of her return

The New Dawn

Hope…
A new dawn crests the horizon.
The promise of a new tomorrow
Your light has returned
Winter has turned to spring

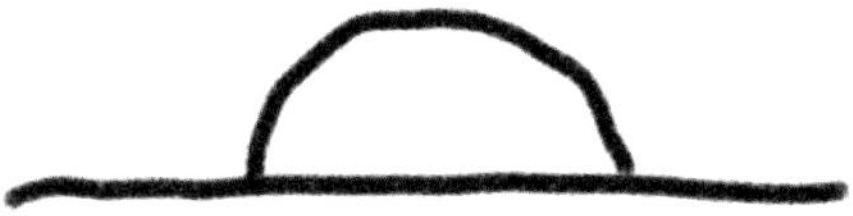

PART I

THE DESCENT

"A down-then-up perspective doesn't fit into our Western philosophy of progress"

RICHARD ROHR
(Franciscan Priest and Writer on Spirituality)

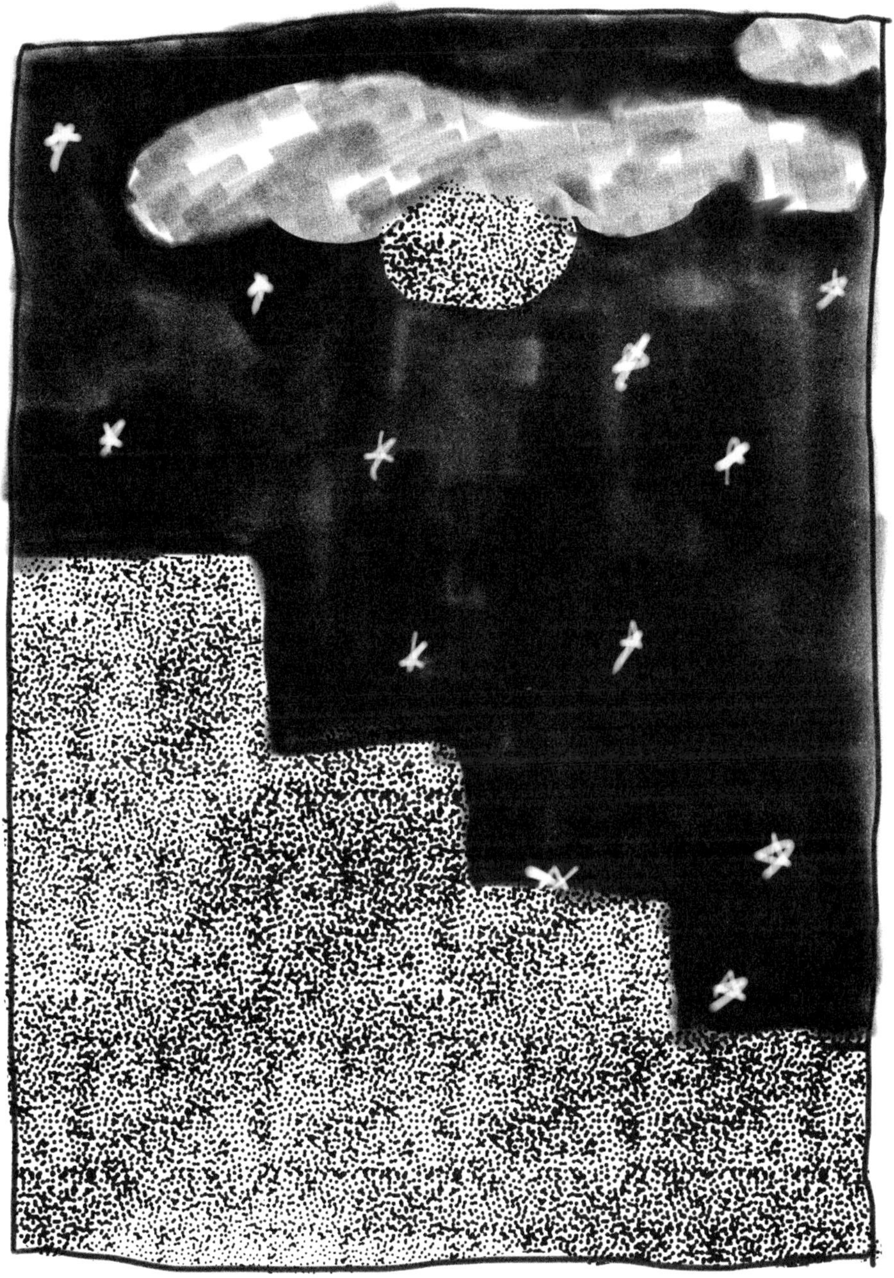

Confusion, Bewilderment and Despair

Confusion, bewilderment, and despair mark this time. Life has changed in an instant. There appears to be no roadmap for the way ahead. All seems lost. All you can do is allow yourself to fall into the oncoming arms of the dark.

The Descent marks the departure from childhood survival mechanisms and the ego's fortifications against pain and vulnerability. From birth well into adulthood, society conditions us to adapt, often at the cost of our authentic selves.

Life's upheavals necessitate internal inquiries to help us address the impact of social conditioning and find new ways forward. Yet, the strong pull of societal norms, along with our ego's protestations to stay 'safe' and repeat the behaviour patterns of the past (despite the ongoing pain), often enforces a surface-level focus that can close our eyes to the need for deeper introspection.

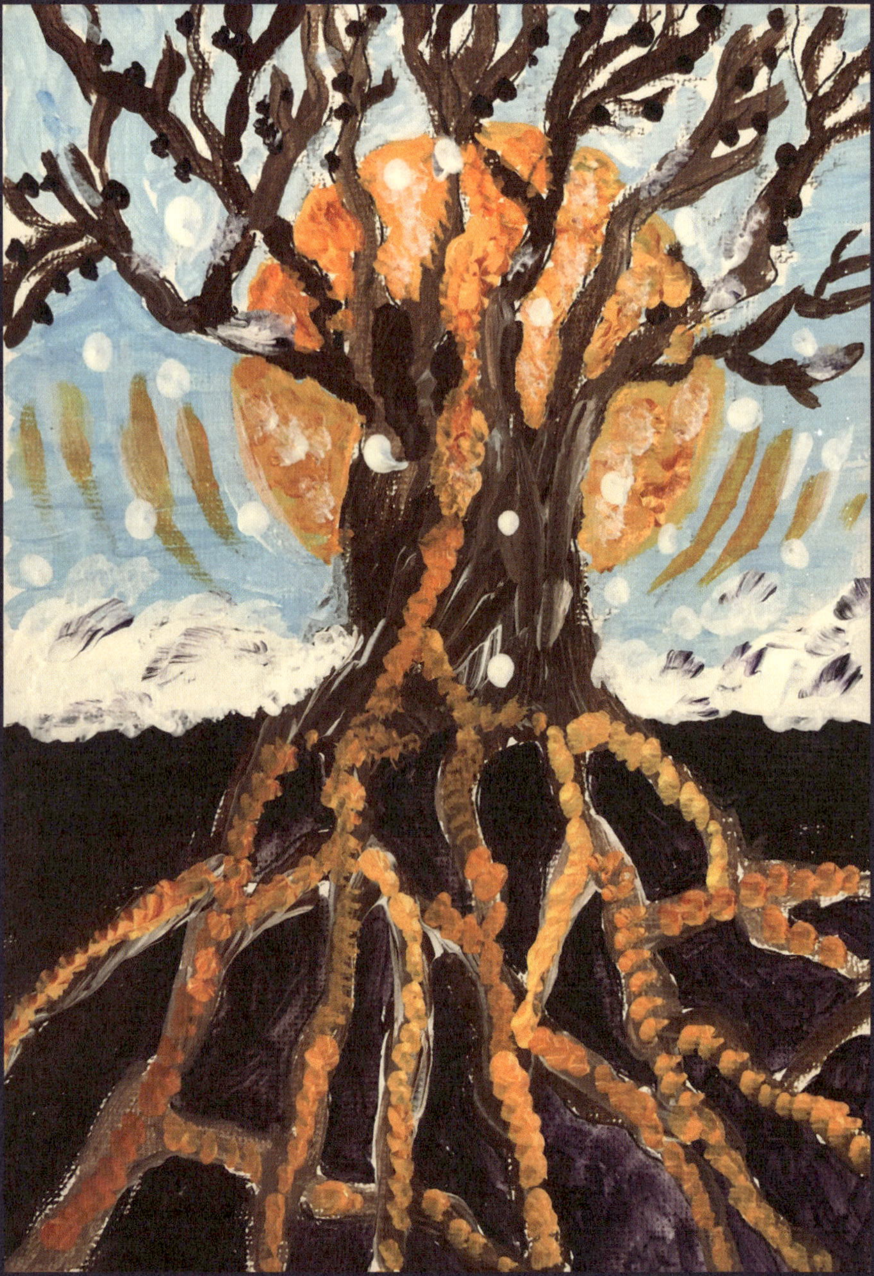

Winter
will take you by
surprise.

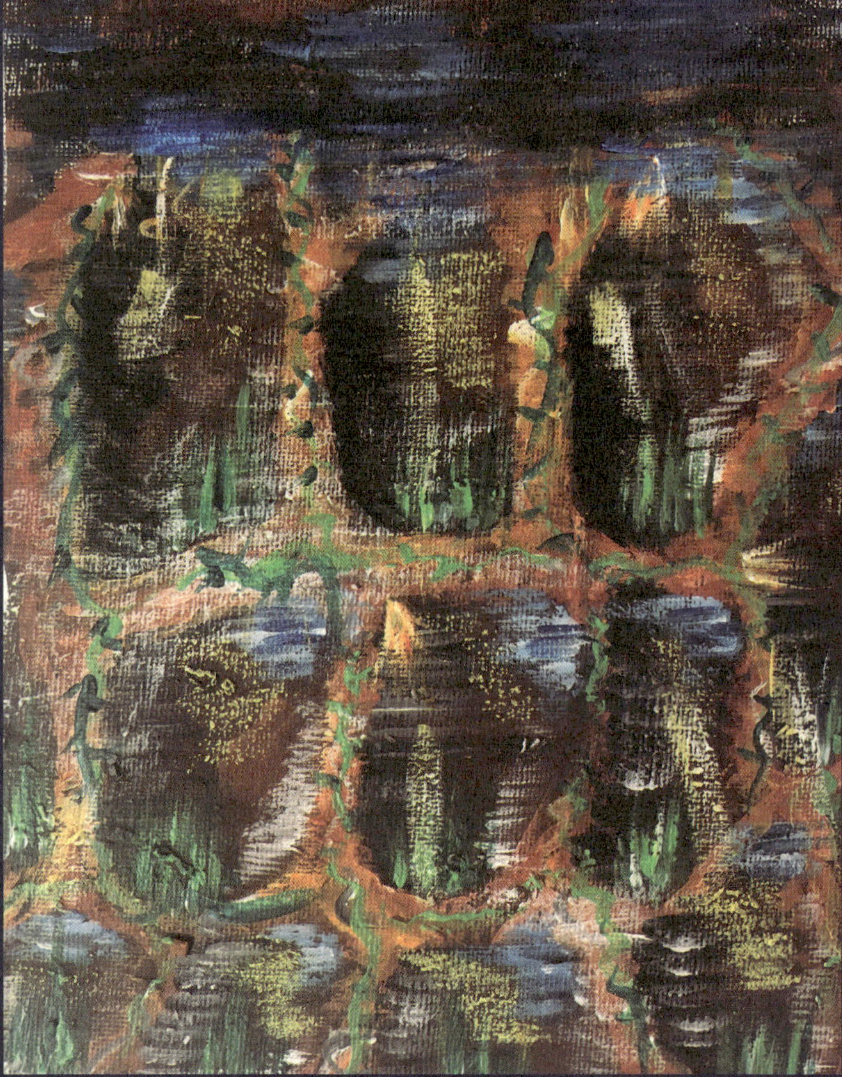